HEAL YOUR SHOULDER

Rotator Cuff Rehabilitation

Kady Dash

CONTENTS

Notice of Rights

INTRODUCTION

I 've made many mistakes after I injured my shoulder because I did not realize how serious the problem was and how long it would take me to recover. This book captures my experience and what I should have done differently, what helped me relieve the pain and ultimately become pain-free.

One of the critical parts of my recovery was physical therapy. I spent many weeks doing supervised physical therapy exercises. This book includes a collection of exercises and instructions that I found to be most effective in my rehabilitation.

THE INJURY

I have worked on the computer every day for over 30 years, having no repetitive motion injuries. I never had shoulder pain before, so when the pain began during an intense work period, I did not stop and kept working to meet a deadline. I was doing a lot of copy and paste motions. Copy and paste motion required me to move my hand left and right with a computer mouse. I was doing this work for over eight hours a day for more than a week.

One night, as I finally met my deadline and went to bed, I could not sleep from the acute pain in my shoulder and neck. The next day, I could not turn my head left or right while driving my car to check for traffic. I was a complete wreck for about three days. In three or four days, using an over-the-counter anti-inflammatory medication, I graduated from being in agony to having intense pain, which got more acute each time I worked on a computer for more than a few minutes.

I took several vacation days so I could stop using my arm for typing altogether. I got a different mousing device to change the angle of my hand. Rest and a different mousing device helped a little.

I continued to take over the counter anti-inflammatory pills (aspirin was particularly helpful), but the pain did not go away. I kept telling myself that it will get better soon, but nine months later, I still had pain at the top of the shoulder, in the back of the neck, and the bicep area from the shoulder to the elbow.

VISIT WITH THE SPECIALIST

After nine months of pain, I decided to see an orthopedic specialist. The exam started with the doctor collecting information about the history of my injury. During the exam, the doctor checked the range of motion of my shoulder and muscle strength. We also talked about what movements make my shoulder hurt.

The doctor performed two tests: an X-ray to check for fractures of the bones and an ultrasound to check for tears in the tendons, muscles, and bursas in my shoulder.

The X-ray images showed the parts of the body in different shades of black and white. Different tissues absorbed different amounts of radiation. Calcium in bones absorbs x-rays the most, so bones looked white. Fat and other soft tissues absorb less and looked gray. Air absorbed the least radiation, so areas with air looked black. If there were a break in the bone, it would appear as a black line on the white space. The X-ray also can show bone spurs and arthritis, which can cause muscle irritation and inflammation.

The ultrasound uses high-frequency sound waves to produce images of structures within the body. During an ultrasound, the doctor applied gel to my skin over the area being examined. The gel helped prevent air pockets, which can block the sound waves that create the images. The gel was water-based, and it was easy to remove after the exam by just wiping the area with a tissue.

During the test, the doctor pressed a small, hand-held transducer against my shoulder and moved it around the entire shoulder area. The transducer sent sound waves into my body, collected the waves that bounced back and sent them to a computer to display them. Ultrasound was painless, and sound waves are very safe; no worry about any side effects.

Fortunately for me, the tests showed no breaks or tears.

WHAT IS A ROTATOR CUFF

A rotator cuff is a group of four muscles and tendons that surround the shoulder joint. They keep the head of the upper arm bone firmly within the shallow socket of the shoulder.

The first image below shows a normal shoulder structure; the second image shows an inflamed rotator cuff.

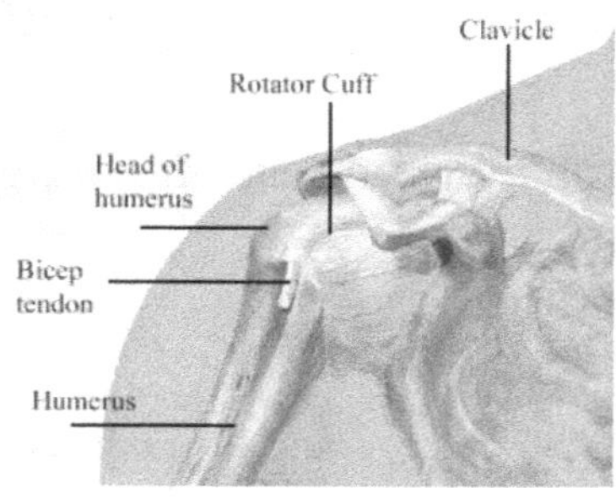

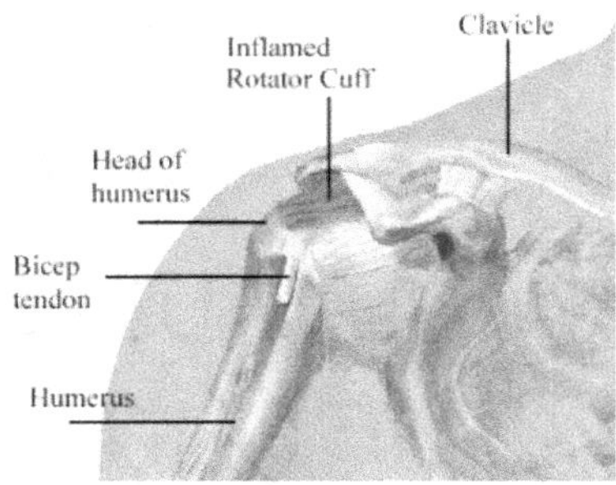
Inflamed
Rotator Cuff
Clavicle
Head of
humerus
Bicep
tendon
Humerus

WHAT CAUSED
THE PAIN

The doctor explained that my pain was caused by swelling, which resulted from the over-use of the shoulder joint. The swelling caused the pinching of the tendons in the shoulder. The pain in the bicep area, the doctor said, was referred pain from the bicep tendon pinched in the shoulder joint and this pain is very frequently associated with rotator cuff injuries.

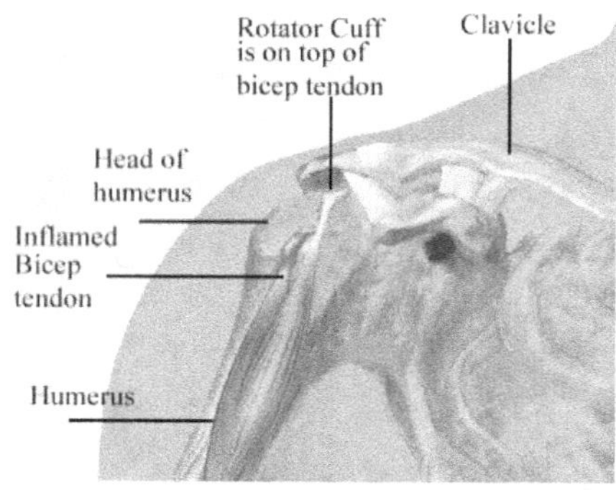

DO NOT IGNORE THE PAIN

Without treatment, rotator cuff problems may lead to permanent loss of motion or weakness and may cause progressive shoulder joint degeneration. Although resting the shoulder is necessary for recovery, keeping the shoulder immobilized for a prolonged time can cause the connective tissue enclosing the joint to become thickened and tight (also known as the frozen shoulder).

CORTISONE SHOT

With no breaks or tears, the doctor gave me a two-step solution to healing my shoulder. The first step was a cortisone shot, and the second step was a prescription for physical therapy. He told me that if I did not feel significantly better in six months, I could come back for another cortisone shot.

Cortisone shots are injections that can help relieve pain and inflammation in a specific area of your body. Cortisone shot reduces inflammation, and this reduces the chances of the muscles being pinched by the shoulder joint. The shot typically reduces swelling by 80%, and physical therapy often helps with the rest. A repeat cortisone shot in six months often is used for stubborn cases. Because of the potential side effects, the number of shots you can get in a year is limited. Repeated cortisone shots might damage the cartilage within a joint.

The doctors typically limit the number of cortisone injections to no more often than every six weeks, and usually not more than three or four times a year.

The injections usually contain a corticosteroid medication and a local anesthetic. The corticosteroid medication relieves pain and inflammation over time, and an anesthetic to provide immediate pain relief.

The doctor gave me the cortisone shot during the first visit. I had to change into an examination gown. The injection area was at the top of my shoulder in the back. The doctor started by cleaning that area, then rubbed the local anesthetic to numb the area where the needle would be inserted, then, finally, injecting the shot. I did not feel any pain, only pressure from the needle being inserted. The medication was then released into the injection site. The doctor told me to watch for any signs of infection, visible as redness and swelling around the injection area. He said that taking showers was okay, but I should not take hot bath soaks or whirlpool for two days. He warned me that some people have redness and a feeling of warmth in the chest and face after a cortisone shot. I had a little redness around the area where the needle was inserted, but no warmth or other side effects.

Cortisone shots commonly cause a temporary flare-up in pain and inflammation for up to 48 hours after the injection. After that, the affected joint's pain and inflammation should decrease and can last up to several months.

I noticed the cortisone shot began having an effect in a couple of days. Even though the pain was still there, it was significantly dulled. I had no flair-up in pain that the doctor warned me about. The pain continued to decrease over the next four weeks. The effects of a cortisone shot can last several months. During this time, the damaged tissues heal, and when the shot wears out, the pain often does not return.

A few months after the shot, I still had some pain in the shoulder, but it was significantly less severe than before, and my shoulder continued to slowly get better during the next six or seven months.

PHYSICAL THERAPY

In a couple of weeks after the cortisone shot, I began physical therapy. My physical therapy regimen was two sessions a week for eight weeks at the cost of $80 per session. In addition to in-person sessions, I had to do a set of daily exercises at home. I include these exercises in the following chapters.

The most valuable part of the physical therapy visits was a hands-on massage of the knotted muscles around my shoulder and neck. The massage portion of physical therapy only lasted for a few minutes but provided hours of pain relief.

PHYSICAL THERAPY: MASSAGE

I thought I would not be able to find a substitute for these hands-on massage sessions when I stopped going to physical therapy, but I was able to find a substitute that worked just as well and only cost me around $10. What is this magic tool? A plain Lacrosse ball that I pressed against the wall and rolled around with my back and shoulder. As soon as the ball pressed against a knotted muscle in my back, it was more painful, but as I continued to roll the ball over that area, the pain dissipated. To find all tender areas, I change the shoulder and hand position slightly as I rolled the ball into tender spots.

Lacrosse ball massage worked just like a physical therapy specialist's firm hand. What was better than the hands-on therapy was that I could do it several times a day as soon as I felt the pain in my shoulder.

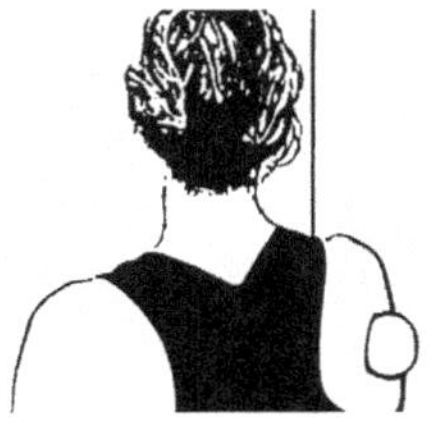

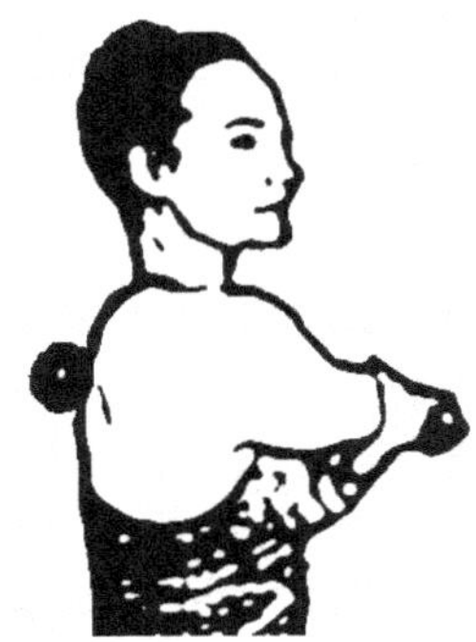

I feel that these acupressure sessions several times a day were the second major turning point (second only to the cortisone shot) on my road to recovery. As soon as I felt a twinge of pain, I could reduce it or eliminate it by massaging the muscle that was beginning to tense up.

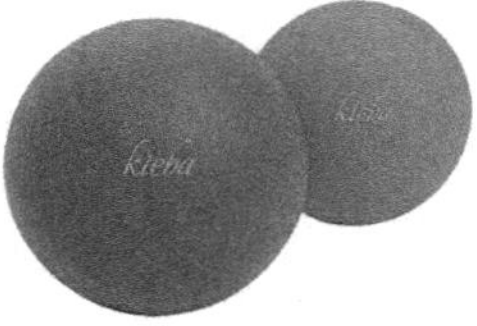

The Lacrosse balls have just the right firmness for the massage. They are hard, but they also have a little bit of a give. After I discovered Lacrosse balls, I tried a few other balls for comparison. I found that plastic balls were too hard and thus too painful, tennis balls did not roll as well, their fuzzy surface generated more friction with the wall, and softer balls did not provide enough firmness to generate enough pressure on the tight muscle to make a difference. You can buy Lacrosse balls on Amazon for under $10. Note that there are balls sold under the massage balls label for more money, but it is just a marketing technique. I purchased several of them for comparison and they turned out to be exactly the same as the Lacrosse balls.

PHYSICAL THERAPY: HEAT AND COLD

Shoulder physical therapy exercises can be performed using inexpensive and simple exercise tools.

My in-person physical therapy sessions always started with applying heat to my shoulder. In my at-home sessions, I continued the same routine. Before exercise, I applied heat to both the front and back of the shoulder for 10 minutes. I started by using an electric heating pad and later purchased a moist heat pad.

A moist heat pad is a pad filled with clay. In the physical therapy office, this clay pad was heated by placing it in a basin filled with hot water. A home version of the pad is heated by placing it in the microwave. My physical therapy instructor said that she found moist heat pads more effective because clay provides even heat over the pad's entire surface.

Electric heating pads produce a "dry heat." Dry heat absorbs moisture from the skin, which can contribute to discomfort. Moist heat therapy has a wet heat source. This could include hot water bottle, steam towels, hot baths, or moist heated clay packs.

When I finished the exercises, I used a cold compress to cool the muscles. I started by usung a few ACE bandages that were kept in the freezer. I taped them to my shoulder with a self-adhesive bandage. A few weeks later, I purchased a cold pack designed to fit around the shoulders. The benefit of a shoulder pack is that it does not need to be taped. Its shape is designed like the top of a shirt and rests on your shoulders, and has a snap closure on the front, which keeps it in place. It was comfortable enough that I could work on the computer while the ice pack rested on shoulders.

PHYSICAL THERAPY: RESISTANCE BANDS

I used resistance bands every day. They are inexpensive, easy to take along even when I travel, and enhance both the exercise's quality and variety. Resistance bands come in different resistance strengths and different shapes. Some are long strips; others are rubber loops; some are rubber ropes with handles. My physical therapy instructor preferred long latex elastics bands on which she added knots for attaching them to the doorjamb.

Rubber loops also come in various lengths (short ones are around 12" and long ones are around 5-7 feet).

I found the long strips the most universal because they can be knotted to make them shorter if an exercise calls for a shorter length. There are many options for these bands available on Amazon. You can narrow down your search by searching for "resistance bands 5 feet", which will return the longer ones. I used different resistances based on the exercise and on my overall fitness level as my abilities improved with time. The resistance bands are color-coded, and different colors mean different resistance strengths. There is no one common standard used by all manufacturers. The most common color coding is this: yellow bands have the least resistance, medium bands are typically green or red, blue bands provide strong resistance, and extra heavy resistance bands are typically black.

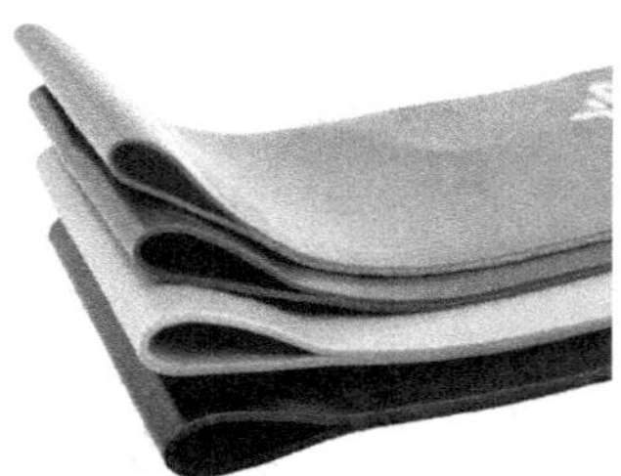

My physical therapy instructor started my exercise regimen with red bands, and a few weeks later, I graduated to green bands, which provide somewhat more resistance.

The straps are made out of thin rubber material that becomes brittle with time. I replace the straps every year. If you don't replace them, they eventually become so brittle that they break up into small chunks. This happened to my first set of resistance bands before I realized they don't last forever. The rubber chunks made quite a mess to clean up, and now I avoid this problem by replacing them once a year.

SHOULDER PAIN EXERCISES

SCAPULAR RETRACTION BILATERAL EXERCISE

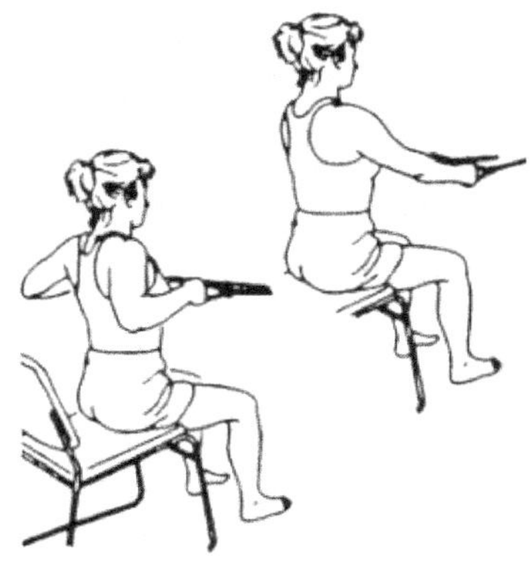

Scapular Retraction Bilateral exercise uses three feet, a green resistance band, with a knot in the center.

- Anchor the knot in the door frame.
- Facing the anchor, pull arms back, bring shoulder blades together.
- Do not raise shoulders.

- Keep elbows close to the body.
- You can do this exercise standing up or sitting on a non-rolling chair.
- Move slowly.
- Repeat exercise 10 times per set.
- Do three sets per session.
- You can pause between each set or continue whatever feels comfortable.
- The exercise should cause no pain. Your muscles may feel tired but not in pain. If you feel pain, stop.
- Do this exercise once a day.

SHOULDER STRENGTHENING USING RESISTED EXTENSION

This exercise uses a three-foot red resistance band. One side of the band has a knot to use as an anchor; the other end has a loop to put your hand through.

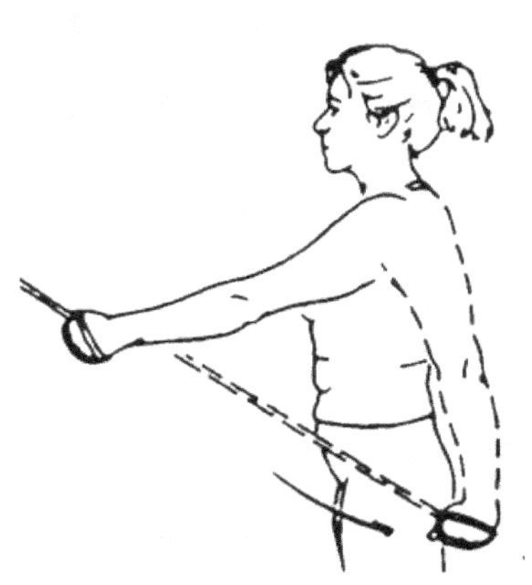

- Anchor the band in a door frame.
- Hold the resistance band in the right hand with the arm forward.
- Pull arm back, keeping the elbow straight until it is just past vertical.
- Move your arm slowly, without pauses.
- Repeat this exercise ten times per set.
- Do three sets per session.
- You can pause between sets or continue without stopping whatever feels comfortable.
- The exercise should cause no pain. Your muscles may feel tired but not in pain. If you feel pain, stop. Do this exercise once a day.

SHOULDER RESISTED EXTERNAL ROTATION IN NEUTRAL BILATERAL

This exercise is performed using two feet red band with a knot at each end of the band. The two knots make it easier to hold the band, so it does not slip out of your hands. This exercise can be performed sitting or standing.

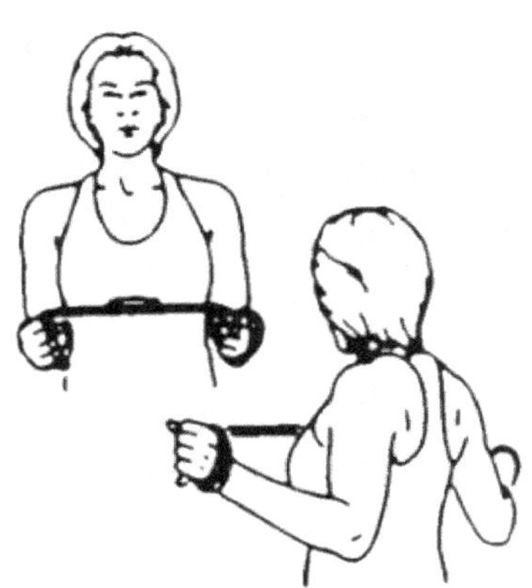

- Hold the hands bent at elbows 90 degrees, elbows touching the torso, with forearms forward.

- Your thumbs should be up.

- Move hands away from each other.

- Pinch your shoulder blades and rotate forearms out.

- Another variation of this exercise is to hold hands with the thumbs out; however, you must avoid holding the bands with the thumbs pointing inwards to face each other.

- Repeat this exercise ten times per set.

- Do two sets per session.

- You can pause between sets or continue without stopping whatever feels comfortable. The exercise should cause no pain.

- Your muscles may feel tired but not in pain. If you feel pain, stop.

- Do this exercise once a day.

FLEXIBILITY
DOORWAY STRETCH

Standing in the doorway or corner with hands just below shoulder level and feet in the middle of the doorway.

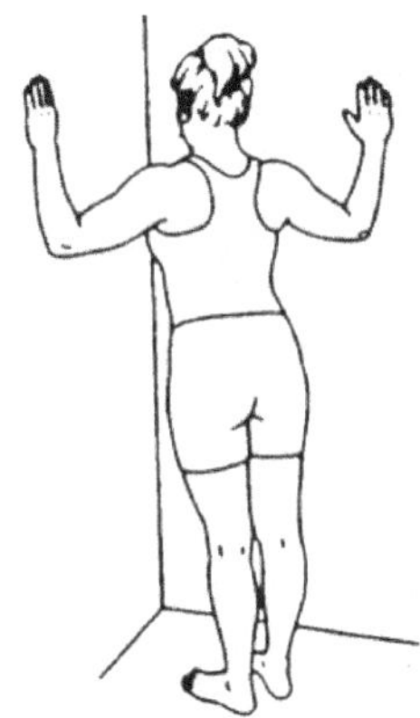

- Step forward until a comfortable stretch is felt across the chest.

- Hold this stretch for 30 seconds.

- Step back.

- Then step forward with another foot.
- Repeat this exercise four times per set.
- Do two sets per session.
- You can pause between sets or continue without stopping whatever feels comfortable.
- The exercise should cause no pain. Your muscles may feel tired but not in pain. If you feel pain, stop. Do this exercise once a day.

RESISTED INTERNAL ROTATION

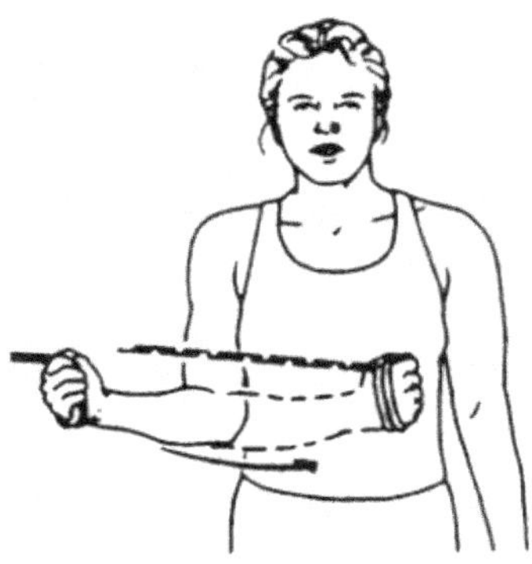

- Hold tubing in the right hand, elbow at the side, and forearm out.

- Rotate forearm across the body.

- Do not raise shoulders.

- Keep elbows close to the body.

- Repeat this exercise ten times per set.

- Do three sets per session.

- You can pause between sets or continue without stopping whatever feels comfortable.

- The exercise should cause no pain. Your muscles may feel tired but not in pain. If you feel pain, stop. Do this exercise once a day.

RESISTED EXTERNAL ROTATION

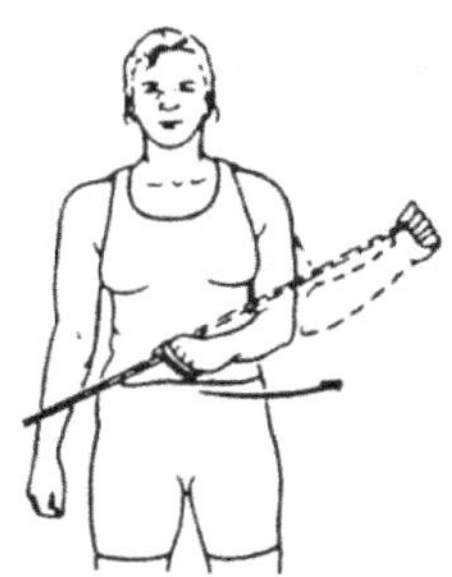

- Hold tubing in the right hand, elbow at the side, and forearm across the body.

- Rotate forearm out.

- Do not raise shoulders.

- Keep elbows close to the body.

- Repeat this exercise ten times per set.

- Do three sets per session.

- You can pause between sets or continue without stopping whatever feels comfortable.

- The exercise should cause no pain. Your muscles may feel tired but not in pain. If you feel pain, stop. Do this exercise once a day.

SCAPULAR: PROTRACTION 90 DEGREE OF FLEXION

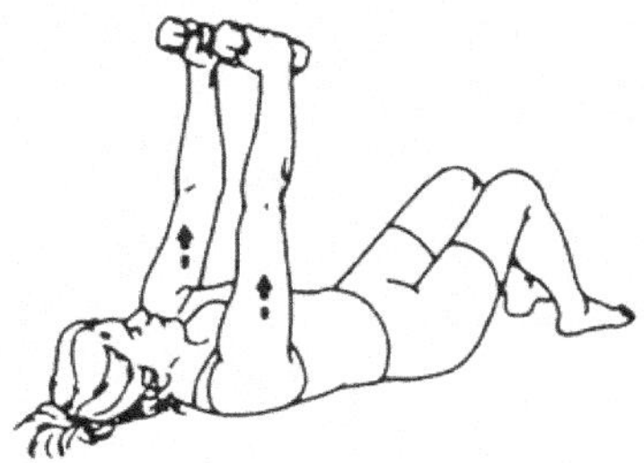

- Holding 1 pound weights, attempt to push arms up towards the ceiling.
- Keep elbows straight and back against the floor.
- When 1 pound weights feel too light, increase the weight to 3/5 pounds.
- Rotate forearm out.
- Repeat this exercise ten times per set.

- Do three sets per session.

- You can pause between sets or continue without stopping whatever feels comfortable.

- The exercise should cause no pain. Your muscles may feel tired but not in pain. If you feel pain, stop. Do this exercise once a day.

NECK PAIN EXERCISES

The neck muscles are often involved in shoulder injuries. To alleviate pain in the neck, muscle trapezius stretch and neck stretch exercises are helpful.

UPPER TRAPEZIUS STRETCH

For the pain on the right-hand side of the neck associated with the right shoulder injury:

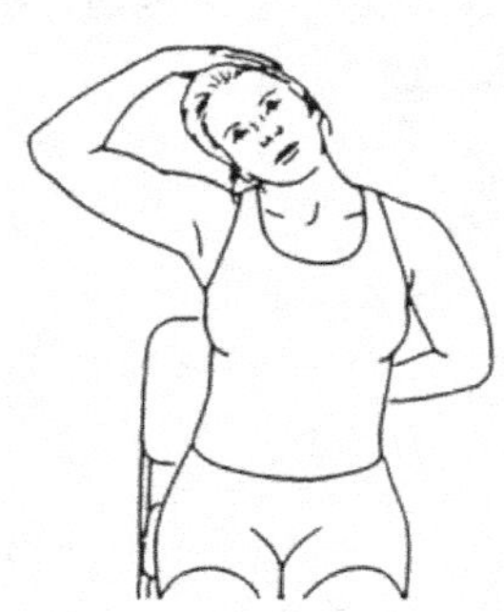

- Gently grasp the head's right side while reaching behind the back with the other hand.
- Then tilt your head towards the left shoulder until a gentle stretch is felt in the neck.
- Try tilting the head slightly forward to stretch the muscle in the back of the neck

on the right-hand side.

NECK STRETCH

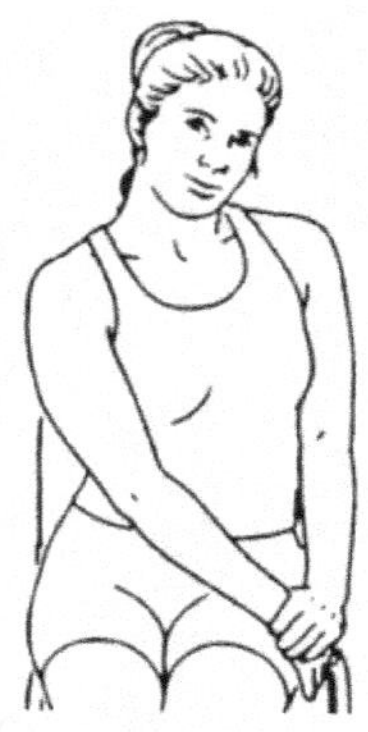

- Sit or Stand

- Grasp the right arm above the wrist and pull down across the body while gently tilting the head in the same direction (i.e., towards the left shoulder).

- Try tilting the head slightly forward to stretch the muscle in the back of the neck on the right-hand side.

PREVENTING THE SHOULDER INJURIES

J ust about everyone is vulnerable to a shoulder injury, even a humble office worker. Daily shoulder stretches and strengthening exercises can help prevent these injuries.

Most people exercise the chest, shoulder, and upper arm's front muscles, but it is equally important to strengthen the muscles in the back of the shoulder and around the shoulder blade to optimize shoulder muscle balance.

Even when my pain decreased to almost noticeable, I continued to do these simple exercises daily. I am also never too far away from my Lacrosse ball (I have one at work and one at home).

It took me about a year to get my shoulder back to the pre-injury pain-free state. I did not need to get the second steroid shot. I needed time, the Lacrosse ball, and physical therapy with rubber bands to heal my shoulder. This book contains my daily routine that keeps my shoulder healthy and pain-free at the cost of only a few minutes every day. If you are reading this book, you are likely to have some shoulder pain. I hope my experience will help you feel better.

If you found this book helpful, I would appreciate it if you would leave a book review.

www.ingramcontent.com/pod-product-compliance
Lightning Source LLC
Chambersburg PA
CBHW061739250726
48657CB00002B/999